Kava Kava, Valerian and Other Nervine Herbs

DEANNE TENNEY

Woodland Publishing
Pleasant Grove, UT

Woodland Publishing, Inc.
P.O. Box 160
Pleasant Grove, UT
84062

Table of Contents

Introduction

In these modern times, most people operate at full speed but are still under constant pressure to do more. Money pressures, lack of time, problems at work, neverending traffic, crying children, family responsibilities—there are many everyday situations that exert great stress on the body and the mind. Some of the symptoms associated with stress include anxiety, depression, irritability, insomnia, illness, stomach tightness, nausea, increased blood pressure, poor concentration, and withdrawal from family and friends.

Stress in itself is not always bad. Some anxiety is normal, and in fact healthy, but a constant, prolonged state of anxiety can lead to mental and physical problems. Individuals react differently to stress, and stress-related medical and emotional problems have increased in the last few decades. A major side effect of these problems is evidenced by the statistic that during the course of a year, more than half of the U.S. population will have difficulty falling asleep. About 33 percent of the population experiences insomnia on a regular basis.[1] Along with anxiety and insomnia, depression is major problem in modern society. Antidepressant medications are commonly prescribed to help people cope with everyday life.

How can we deal with stress and its side effects? How can we reduce the negative results that come from an anxious day at work followed by a restless, near sleepless night? Of course, there are many ways to try and alleviate stress. Countless books, classes and seminars teach us how to get organized, make goals, and streamline our lives. Exercise and meditation are also recognized as helpful to stress management. This booklet will deal with an often overlooked therapy for dealing with any sort of nervous condition—the therapy that involves supplementing a healthy diet with herbs that will strengthen and enhance a person's nervous system. When our nervous system is healthy, we can deal with stress in a positive and healthy way.

Our nervous system is directly related to our immune system. An insufficient immune function can cause the nervous system to work poorly. A lack of essential nutrients can cause the immune system to be weakened and put a strain on the adrenal and thymus glands. This in turn can make the body less able to cope with emotional and physical stress. The question is how to continue living a busy and demanding life and still cope with stress effectively.

One of the first things anyone can do is to make sure they have good eating habits. A healthy diet is a must to help restore strength to the immune and nervous systems. Whole grains, fruits, vegetables, beans, lentils, raw seeds and nuts can help the body stay healthy. Nutritional supplements are also available that can help strengthen the nervous system to help the body deal with stress and emotional problems.

Another way to assist your body in coping with stress is to use the herbs known as nervine herbs. They provide nutrients required by the nervous system, nutrients which strengthen and help the system to heal itself when necessary. Valerian, for example, can help induce a deep and restful sleep—something which can help anyone feel calmer and improve the ability to concentrate and focus on a task. Along with a good diet, nervine herbs and herbal formulas can aid in the performance of the nervous system's essential functions. A healthy nervous system is one very important component of a healthy lifestyle.

KAVA KAVA

(*Piper methysticum*)

Polynesia, Micronesia, Melanesia and many other island communities in the Pacific have traditionally used kava kava in their ceremonial drinks as a mild sedative and relaxant. It is still used today to relax the body and mind and promote a restful sleep. Kava kava is now generally considered an important herb for insomnia and other nervous conditions, as well as being beneficial for pain relief.

Drinking from 100 to 150 ml of kava tea is enough to put most people into a deep, dreamless sleep within thirty minutes. Unlike alcohol and other sedatives, the use of kava does not result in any morning hangover. The kava drinker usually awakens having fully recovered normal physical and mental capacities.[2] Individuals who drink smaller amounts of kava kava express a sense of tranquillity, sociability, and contentment.[3]

The herb's chemical constituents work together so that kava kava can function as an anesthetic, analgesic, anticonvulsive, antifungal and sleep inducer.[4] Research done with animals verifies that kava kava contains anticonvulsant and muscle-relaxing properties.[5] Michael Murray, a well-known naturopathic physician, explains that the key components of kava kava, kavalactones, "appear to act primarily on the limbic system—an ancient part of the brain that affects all other brain activities and is the principal seat of the emotions."[6] Perhaps kava promotes sleep and relaxation by altering the way in which the limbic system influences emotional processes.

Because of its tremendous abilities, kava kava is considered to be one of the most powerful of the herbal muscles relaxants. It is recommended for rheumatism, insomnia, and to relax the body. It has antiseptic properties to help with bladder infections and may be applied directly to wounds.

A huge benefit of kava kava is that, unlike synthetic drugs often prescribed for anxiety and insomnia, it does not seem to lose effectiveness over time.[7] In fact, because of its ability to relax and induce sleep, a recent study showed kava kava to be of significant benefit for people suffering from anxiety.[8] Another study looked at the effects of kava kava on women suffering from menopause. Two groups of twenty women with menopause-related symptoms were treated for eight weeks, one group being given kava kava three times daily and the other group given a placebo. After only one week, the women taking kava kava demonstrated significant improvement. Not only were stress and anxiety reduced, but women reported their general mood as being much better and symptoms of menopause much less noticeable. No side effects were noted.[9]

The effects of kava kava prove it to be an excellent nervine herb. To naturally promote a sense of well-being and contentment is an ability that cannot go unappreciated in the busy, stressful world in which we live.

VALERIAN

(*Valeriana officinalis*)

Ancient Greeks used valerian for digestion, nausea, and urinary tract disorders. Galen, a famous Greek physician, also prescribed valerian as a decongestant. In 1597, herbalist John Gerard recommended this herb for chest congestion, convulsions, and bruises. Native Americans traditionally used valerian for healing wounds. It was accepted in the *U.S. Pharmacopoeia* as a tranquilizer from 1820 until 1942 and was so listed in the *National Formulary* until 1950.

Studies have identified one of the most valuable properties of valerian—the ability to produce a deep, satisfying sleep. The herb acts as a relaxant and is an effective remedy for insomnia.[10] The active ingredients found in valerian root are responsible for relaxing the smooth muscle tissue and depressing the central nervous system. It appears that no single component of the valerian is responsible for all of its sedative activity, but several of the constituents work together.[11] The herb works similar to other standard sleep aids often prescribed, but its advantage lies in the fact that it does not cause the morning grogginess often associated with prescription sleep medications.[12]

Many different studies have confirmed the benefits of valerian for insomnia, anxiety and stress. It is useful for all kinds of sleep disorders, especially when they are related to anxiety, nervousness, headache pain, or physical and mental exhaustion. Research has found valerian to be effective not only in treating insomnia, but also in reducing sleep latency and night awakenings.[13]

Valerian is beneficial for the heart, lungs, liver, stomach, as well as the nerves and the brain. It may also help with epilepsy, hysteria, migraines, and the elimination of worms because it works to calm anxiety, muscle spasms, and nervous tension. Along with the ability to relax and calm, valerian also helps to improve mental acuity and coordination. One study found that hyperactive individuals using valerian were able to concentrate for longer periods of time.[14]

This herb is rich in calcium, which accounts for its ability to strengthen the spine, nerves and brain. It is also high in magnesium and manganese, minerals that works with calcium for healthy bones and nervous system, and selenium, which strengthens the body against immune related disorders. Valerian's niacin content helps prevent cholesterol build-up, irritability, depression, loss of memory and weakness. This herb also contains potassium, iron, sodium, zinc, silicon, vitamins A and C. Valerian is thought to be safe and there appear to be no contraindications to its use even during pregnancy and lactation. It is usually recommended for short-term use.[15]

St. John's Wort

(*Hypericum Perforatum*)

St. John's wort has recently emerged as an herb known to aid the nervous system. Some naturopathic physicians rank kava kava, valerian, St. John's wort, passionflower and hops as the most effective herbs to treat insomnia.[16] A 1994 study published in the *Journal of Geriatric Pyschiatry and Neurology* showed that extracts of St. John's wort gave the benefit of increased deep sleep during the total sleeping period of the patients. The study also makes an interesting connection between sleep and depression; that being many standard antidepressants and MAO inhibitors used to treat people who suffer from depression cause a decrease in deep sleep. St. John's wort has shown great promise in treating both insomnia and depression.[17]

HOPS
(*Humulus lupulus*)

Hops is an herb found commonly throughout the world. It was originally used as a food, the tips being cooked and eaten. Only the young plants were eaten because the older were too tough. Gerarde, a famous herbalist, recommended using the buds in salads. The Romans anciently used hops as a food and Native American tribes found hops to be of great value. Specifically, the Mohicans used it as a sedative and for toothaches and the Menominee tribe used it as a cure-all.

Hops has long been appreciated for its nervine properties. Around 1500, when hops began to be used as a beer ingredient in England, hops farmers noticed that their farmhands often seemed tired and fatigued easily. With time, the herb gained a great reputation as a sedative.[18] During the reign of King George, pillows were filled with hops to promote rest and relaxation when recovering from an illness.

Lupulin, a compound found in hops, is described as a sedative and hypnotic drug and was recognized in the *U.S. Pharmacopoeia* from 1831 to 1916. Modern studies verify that hops indeed has sedative properties. Certain constituents of the plant have been found to contain sedative and hypnotic effects.[19] It is known to be fast-acting, soothing and calming on the nervous system, and is another of the nervine herbs that aids in promoting sleep.[20, 21] Its main uses are to alleviate nervous tension and promote a restful sleep. Hops is also used for its anti-spasmodic effects.[22] Its relaxing effect helps to calm the nerves as well as the muscles in cases of muscle spasms.

This herb is also thought to contain appetizing and tonic properties. It acts as a stimulant to the glands and muscles of the stomach and calms the hyperexcitable gastric nerves. It also has a relaxing influence upon the liver and gall duct, and a laxative effect on the bowels.

Along with its other uses, hops is also used for its antibiotic properties. It is beneficial for sore throats, bronchitis, infections, high fevers, delirium, toothaches, earaches, and pain. A poultice of hops is recommended for inflammation, boils, tumors, and swelling.

Hops is very high in B-complex vitamins, known for their calming effect on the nervous system. They also promote energy and aid in problems of depression, anxiety, nervousness, and memory. Hops is also rich in potassium, which is necessary for nerve transmission, contraction of the muscles, and hormone secretion. Low levels of potassium have been found in people with high blood pressure. Hops also contains magnesium, zinc, copper, iodine, manganese, iron, sodium, and fluoride.

PASSIONFLOWER

(*Passiflora incarnata*)

Passionflower has long been appreciated for its nervine properties. It is known that the Aztecs used it as a sedative and for pain. It was listed in the *National Formulary* as a sedative from 1916 to 1936.

Research on passionflower has found it useful for insomnia, fatigue, spasms and nervous tension.[23] Most of the research done has focused on the herb's sedative action with good results.[24] Studies have shown extract of passionflower to reduce locomotor activity and prolong sleeping.[25] Some tests indicate the use of this herb for pain relief as well as for its sedative effects.[26] It contains anti-inflammatory properties which may be useful for those suffering from arthritis.[27] The active ingredient of the plant is thought to be passiflorine which has similar principles to morphine.[28] Dr. R. Swinburne Clymer, M.D. even refers to passionflower as the nonpoisonous, safe opium of the natural physician.

Passionflower is very soothing to the nervous system and good for hysteria, anxiety, and hyperactivity. It depresses the central nervous system and may be useful in lowering high blood pressure. Herbal combinations containing valerian and passionflower are considered very useful as natural tranquilizers. Passionflower contains calcium and magnesium, both essential for the nervous system. It is safe for both children and the elderly.

VITAMIN B3
(Niacinamide or Niacin)

Vitamin B3 is needed for healthy circulation and gastrointestinal function. It is also necessary for a healthy nervous system. Deficiencies may cause skin problems, diarrhea, apprehension, anxiety, depression, and loss of memory. Vitamin B3 comes in two forms—niacin and niacinamide. Niacin can be converted into niacinamide, and the body is also able to make niacinamide from tryptophan, an amino acid found in animal foods.[29] The problem is that the body only produces a small portion of what it needs.

Vitamin B3 is an important element of the hormonal system. It aids the body in producing cortisone, thyroxine, insulin, and male and female sex hormones. Hormonal problems can affect the nervous system and lead to nervous system disorders and mental problems. This vitamin has been used to treat schizophrenia and autism in children with some success. There are some psychiatric doctors who treat mental disorders with both natural supplements (including niacin) and drugs. Studies have found benefits for the treatment of epilepsy by using niacinamide, along with vitamin E, B-6 and calcium, together with anticonvulsant medication.[30] Vitamin B3 may also help to increase memory and improve mental function.

Along with its influence on the brain and nervous system, niacin also has a beneficial effect on the circulatory system. This can help in the prevention of high cholesterol, high blood pressure, arteriosclerosis, and heart disease.[31] Studies have found that it may also play a role in the prevention of certain types of cancer. It seems to have an effect on some carcinogens. Vitamin B-3 performs many valuable functions in the body and a deficiency can be detrimental.

Inositol

Inositol is a B-vitamin cofactor. It is often found in combinations containing the B-complex vitamins. The level of inositol found in the nerves is fifty times higher than the level found in the blood, so it is obviously important for nervous system function. It seems that its specific action is aiding the conduction of nerve impulses.[32] Inositol has helped individuals with sleep disorders and anxiety, as well as hyperactive children.

Along with choline, inositol is thought to help cleanse the blood of excessive fats and to increase the metabolism of fats. It assists in stimulating the action of the heart and in reducing blood cholesterol levels. Inositol aids the liver in removing fats and is beneficial in helping to prevent hardening of the arteries. It helps to stimulate normal growth patterns and digestive action.

POTASSIUM

When individuals are under stress for long periods of time, they begin to feel so "strung out" that it doesn't take much to exhaust them. Exhaustion may result in a total collapse of body functions or a collapse of specific organs. Prolonged stress puts a huge load on many organ systems.

One of the major causes of exhaustion is the loss of potassium ions. When the cells of the body lose potassium, they function less effectively and eventually die. It is easy to see that it is critical to maintain potassium levels within the body. This can best be done by eating foods rich in potassium and avoiding foods high in sodium. The daily intake of potassium should be at least three to five grams per day. Many vegetables are rich in potassium, especially tomatoes, avocados, lima beans and potatoes. Bananas, peaches and other fresh fruits are rich in potassium, and unprocessed meats and fish are also good sources.[33] Sufficient potassium levels will strengthen the body so that the negative effects of stress will not wear us out and result in exhaustion.

MELATONIN

There has a been a lot of hype recently about the miraculous benefits of melatonin, but many individuals are still not quite sure what it is or what it actually does. Melatonin is a hormone found naturally in the body. It is secreted by the pineal gland and contributes to the setting of the body clock-cycles of night and day. As daylight disappears, the eyes send a signal to the brain which in turn signals the pineal gland to start pumping melatonin. This causes a drop in body temperature, a slowing of the body's metabolism and sleepiness. When sunlight appears, melatonin production slows and the body awakens. This process continues through life, but the secretion of melatonin seems to decrease with age. This may be one contributing factor for increased sleeping problems that occur with age. Melatonin has helped many individuals with sleep disorders who are looking for a natural treatment. Even pharmaceutical companies are rushing to get in on the action by preparing prescription medications using melatonin.

Many studies have been done to test the effectiveness and safety of melatonin. In fact, research has been ongoing for many years. The majority of studies have been done using laboratory animals, but human studies are also ongoing. In one animal study done in 1967 at the National Heart Institute in Bethesda, Maryland, mice were given 800 mg of melatonin per kilogram of body weight.[34] The mice exhibited no significant ill effects.

The researchers would have had to give more melatonin to find the amount that is lethal for fifty percent of the animals (LD 50), but they could not concentrate the melatonin any further in the amount of liquid the mice had to drink. The 800 mg/kg is equivalent to giving an average-sized human over 50,000 mg.[35]

A study reported in the April 1994 issue of *Your Health* studied melatonin in treating insomnia. Subjects were given either a placebo or melatonin and placed in a dark room in the middle of the day. They were asked to close their eyes for thirty minutes. Falling asleep under these circumstances can be difficult. Those given melatonin fell asleep within five to six minutes while those given the placebo took an average of 25 minutes to fall asleep.

These findings are of import for those people who are required to do a lot of traveling. Individuals who travel frequently have used melatonin to ease the problem of jet lag. Sleep patterns, when interrupted, can be a nuisance and cause headaches, fatigue and even lower the immune response. A supplement of melatonin, taken in the evening when in a new time zone is entered, can stimulate the body's own secretion of the hormone and allow the body to adjust to a new sleep cycle. The general recommendation is one mg of melatonin for each hour of time change.

Human studies have revealed no serious side effects when using melatonin. In a few cases some have reported dizziness, bad dreams or slight depression (in those predisposed to this condition). The symptoms subsided as soon as the melatonin supplementation was stopped. Even individuals using high doses have not seemed to suffer from any significant problems.

High doses were thought to be needed in early experiments, but new research seems to indicate that melatonin is useful in much lower amounts—even less than one milligram. Some people have even fallen asleep taking as little as .3 mg of melatonin.[36] Keep in mind that there are no long-term studies and more research is expected which may indicate other results.

There is evidence that melatonin has even more benefits than just helping with sleep and jet lag. There have been studies done which point to its powerful antioxidant and antiaging properties. Some preliminary animal research has pointed to improvements in health and longer lifespan in animal given melatonin supplements. In fact, life was prolonged by about 25 percent in mice treated with melatonin. Further research is also currently being done as to the effect of melatonin on cancer cells. Great results have been noted thus far, and, with time, there will be even more evidence of the benefits of melatonin for serious health ailments.

CONCLUSION

Each of us deal with unique problems and challenges in our daily lives. We also respond to stress and deal with stress in very different ways. Since our jobs, families and relationships are probably not going to suddenly be perfect overnight, it is up to us to learn to manage the stress present in our lives.

Having a healthy nervous system is one of the best ways to deal with stress. Making sure our diet is balanced and rich in vitamins and minerals is a first step to a strong and healthy body. Supplementing with herbs like valerian and kava kava can do a lot to promote rest and relaxation, which makes it much easier to deal with whatever problems come up during the day. Hops, St. John's wort and passionflower are also known to sedate and relax. Vitamin B3, inositol and potassium work to promote the healthy functioning of the nervous system and prevent nervous disorders. And the wonderful effects of melatonin on the nervous system are just beginning to be appreciated. Treating our nervous systems to such supplements will be of benefit to both us and the people we associate with every day.

ENDNOTES

1. Michael T. Murray, N.D. *The Healing Power of Herbs.* Rocklin, CA: Prima Publishing, 1995, p 371
2. Ibid., p. 214.
3. Ibid., p. 213
4. Ibid., p 216.
5. "Kava Kava." *The Lawrence Review of Natural Products.* St. Louis: Facts and Comparisons, May 1987.
6. Murray, p. 214
7. P.H. Duffield and D. Jamieson. "Development of tolerance to Kava in mice." *Clinical Exp Pharmacol Physiology,* 18, 1991, pp5 71-578.
8. James A. Duke. *Handbook of Medicinal Herbs.* Boca Raton, Florida: CRC Press, Inc., 1985, p 381.
9. Murray, p. 216.
10. Ibid., p 196.
11. "Valerian." *The Lawrence Review of Natural Products.* Oct. 1991.
12. *Reader's Digest Family Guide to Natural Medicine.* Pleasantville, N.Y.: The Reader's Digest Association, Inc., 1993, p 325.
13. Donald J. Brown, N.D. "Valerian Root: Non-Addictive Alternative for Insomnia and Anxiety." *Quarterly Review of Natural Medicine.* Fall 1994, p 222.
14. Daniel B. Mowrey. *Herbal Tonic Therapies.* New Canaan, Connecticut: Keats Publishing, Inc., 1993, p 152.
15. Brown, 223.
16. Murray, p. 371.
17. *Journal of Geriatric Psychiatry and Neurology,* 1994, p. S93-94.
18. Michael Castleman. *The Healing Herbs.* St. Martin's

Press, 1991, p. 213.
19. V.E. Tyler. *The Honest Herbal.* Philadelphia: G.F. Stickley Co., 1987, p 176.
20. Daniel B. Mowrey. *The Scientific Validation of Herbs.* New Canaan, Connecticut: Keats Publishing, Inc., 1986, p 217.
21. Michael Murray, N.D. and Joseph Pizzorno, N.D. *Encyclopedia of Natural Medicine.* Rocklin, CA: Prima Publishing, 1991, p 393.
22. Mowrey, *Herbal Tonic Therapies.* p. 181
23. Peter Holmes. *The Energetics of Western Herbs.* Boulder: Artemis Press, 1989, p 656.
24. Mowrey, *Herbal Tonic Therapies.* p 160.
25. Peter R. Bradley. *British Herbal Compendium.* British Herbal Medicine Association, p 172.
26. Mowrey, p 110.
27. Reader's Digest, p 319.
28. Duke, p 347.
29. Shari Lieberman and Nancy Bruning. *The Real Vitamin and Mineral Book.* Garden City Park, N.Y.: Avery Publishing Group Inc., 1990, p 87.
30. Lieberman, 88.
31. Dr. Art Ulene and Dr. Val Ulene. *The Vitamin Strategy.* Berkeley, CA: Ulysses Press, 1994, p 60.
32. Dr. Michael Colgan, *Your Personal Vitamin Profile.* N.Y.: Quill, 1982, 145.
33. Murray, p. 97.
34. Nature, 1967; 214; pp.919-920.
35. Ray Sahelian, M.D., *Let's Live,* October 1995, p 35.
36. Sahelian, p 38